MW00446370

# 'Mudras for Weight-Loss'

## 21 Simple Hand Gestures for Effortless Weight-Loss

# *Advait*

# Disclaimer and FTC Notice

**Mudras for Weight-Loss: 21 Simple Hand Gestures for Effortless Weight-Loss**
Copyright © 2014, Advait. All rights reserved.

**ISBN-13**: 978-1512249163

**ISBN-10**: 1512249165

# Contents

# What are Mudras?

According to the Vedic culture of ancient India, our entire world is made of 'the five elements' called as *The Panch-Maha-Bhuta's*. The five elements being **Earth**, **Water**, **Fire**, **Wind** and **Space/Vacuum**. They are also called the earth element, water element, fire element, wind element and space element.

These five elements constitute the human body – the nutrients from the soil (earth) are absorbed by the plants which we consume (thus we survive on the earth element), the blood flowing through own veins represents the water element, the body heat represents the fire element, the oxygen we inhale and the carbon dioxide we exhale represents the wind element and the sinuses we have in our nose and skull represent the space element.

As long as these five elements in our body are balanced and maintain appropriate levels we remain healthy. An imbalance of these elements in the human body leads to a deteriorated health and diseases.

Now understand this, the command and control center of all these five elements lies in our fingers. So literally, our health lies at our fingertips.

The Mudra healing method that I am going to teach you depends on our fingers.

To understand this, we should first know the finger-element relationship:

Thumb – Fire element.

Index finger – Wind element.

Middle finger – Space/Vacuum element.

Third finger – Earth element.

Small finger – Water element.

This image will give you a better understanding of the concept:

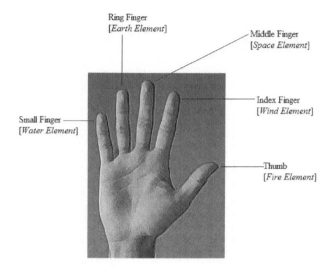

When the fingers are brought together in a specific pattern and are touched to each other, or slightly pressed against each other, the formation is called as a *'Mudra'*.

When the five fingers are touched and pressed in a peculiar way to form a Mudra, it affects the levels of the five elements in our body, thus balancing those elements and inducing good health.

**P.S.** The Mudra Healing Methods aren't just theory or wordplay; these are healing methods from the ancient Indian Vedic culture, proven and tested over ages.

# Important

## *Read this before you read any further*

For the better understanding of the reader, detail images have been provided for every mudra along with the method to perform it.

Most of the Mudras given in this book are to be performed using both your hands, but the Mudras whose images show only one hand performing the Mudra, are to be performed simultaneously on both your hands for the Mudras to have the maximum effect.

# How to Use these Mudras for Effortless Weight-Loss?

'Effortless Weight-Loss' through use of Mudras isn't just about burning the excess fat.

Though shedding the excess fat is the core concept of Weight-Loss, an effective Weight-Loss regimen includes;

a) Methods for losing excess fat.

b) Preparing your internal system for effective digestion and efficient assimilation so that you won't gain weight again once you have shed it.

c) Conditioning your body to curb excessive craving of unhealthy foodstuffs.

d) Developing a strong willpower to carry out the fitness regimen and healthy routines.

e) Building self-confidence so that you are not ashamed of your current physique and are proud of the fact, that you have taken positive steps for achieving fitness and leading a healthy life.

***This book does it all;***

Perform Mudra #1, #2 & #3 for shedding excess fat. (See to it that you perform these 3 Mudras at least 3-5 times a day.)

Perform Mudra #4 through #15 for developing a very good digestive system for proper assimilation of consumed food.

Perform Mudra #16, The *'Tritiiya Vayu Mudra'* for curbing excess craving.

And, perform Mudra #17 through #21 to develop a strong willpower and a rock solid Self-Confidence for completing the weight-loss regimen and leading a healthy life forever.

# Mudras #1

## *Lingamudra / Mudra of Divine Masculine Power*

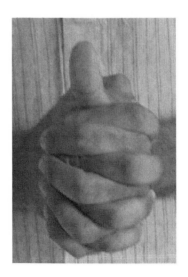

### Method:

This Mudra is to be performed in a sitting position.

Be seated comfortably in an upright posture and concentrate on your breathing to relax.

Clasp the fingers of both of your hands as shown in the image.

Keep the Thumb of your left hand straight and erect.

This Mudra is to be held in front of your abdomen.

(This Mudra is about bringing all the five elements together, with the fire element ruling them all.)


## Duration:

It's a highly effective Mudra, yet a very strong one.

Perform this Mudra for not more than 5-7 minutes at a time.

This Mudra creates a lot of heat in the body, so don't overdo it at once, you can perform multiple sessions of this Mudra, by resting 3-4 minutes between performing this Mudra.


## Uses:

This Mudra reduces laziness and is the most effective Mudra for burning fat.

On a psychological level this Mudra increases your willpower, which is positive enforcement if you are determined to lose weight.

This Mudra also increases ones overall sexual capabilities.

# Mudras #2

## *Rudramudra / Mudra of Lord Shiva*

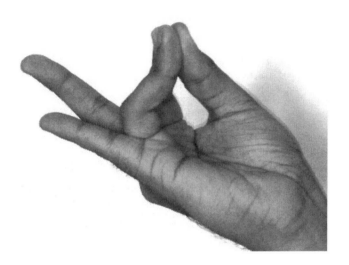

### Method:

This Mudra is to be performed in a sitting position.

Be seated comfortably in an upright posture and concentrate on your breathing to relax.

Place your hands on your thighs with your palms facing upwards.

Touch the tip of your Thumb with the tip of your Index finger and the tip of the Ring finger, press slightly.

Refer the image for more clarity.

## Duration:

This Mudra should be performed for at least 5 minutes and can be performed for 40 minutes at a stretch.

If you are serious about losing weight then this Mudra should be performed at least 4 times a day.

## Uses:

This Mudra reduces sluggishness and is the most effective Mudra for regulating body weight.

It also induces a proper assimilation of the consumed food and works as a good detox Mudra by eliminating toxic fat.

# Mudras #3

## *Suryamudra / Mudra of Sun*

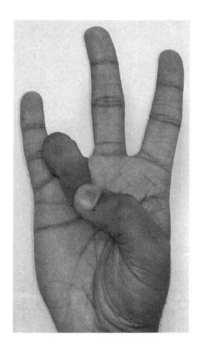

### Method:

This Mudra can be performed while being seated, in a standing position or lying in bed.

Ideally, perform this Mudra in a seating position with your spine kept straight and upright.

Concentrate on your breathing to relax and feel comfortable.

Place your hands on your thighs with your palms facing upwards.

Touch the nail of the Ring finger with the tip of your Thumb and press slightly.

Perform this Mudra for 30 minutes, on an empty stomach, first thing in the morning.

## Duration:

This Mudra should be performed for at least 15 minutes and can be performed for 40 minutes at a stretch.

As advised above, perform it for 30 minutes at a stretch in the morning and then perform this Mudra for at least 4 more times throughout the day, for at least 15 minutes at a time.

## Uses:

This Mudra reduces sluggishness, and is extremely affective in burning excess body fat.

It also detoxifies our body by eliminating toxic fat and cholesterol.

# Mudras #4

## *Apaanmudra / Mudra of Downward Force*

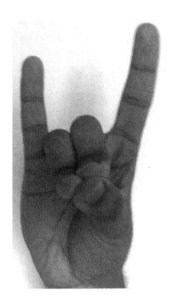

**Method:**

This Mudra is to be performed in a sitting position.

Be seated comfortably in an upright posture and concentrate on your breathing to relax.

Touch the tip of your thumb with the tip of your middle finger and the tip of the ring finger, and press slightly.

Keep the index finger and the Little finger straight as shown in the image.

This Mudra should be performed on both the hands. Rest the hands on your thighs.

See to it that you are completely relaxed while performing this Mudra.

## Duration:

This Mudra should be performed for at least 5 minutes and can be performed for 40 minutes at a stretch.

This Mudra should be performed twice a day, once in the morning and once in the evening for best results.

****Very Important

**DO NOT PERFORM THIS MUDRA DURING PREGNANCY.**

# Mudras #5

## *Chakramudra / Mudra of Wheel*

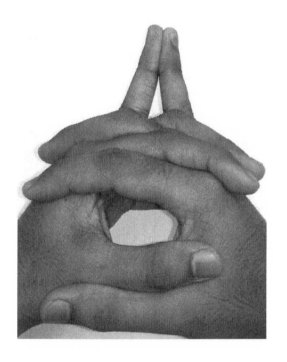

**Method:**

This Mudra is to be performed in a sitting position.

Be seated comfortably in an upright posture and concentrate on your breathing to relax.

Interlace your fingers together as shown in the image.

Extend both your Ring fingers upwards, then touch the tips of these two fingers and press slightly.

This Mudra is to be held in front of your navel.

## Duration:

This Mudra should be performed for at least 5 minutes and can be performed for 40 minutes at a stretch.

This Mudra should be performed twice a day, once in the morning and once in the evening for best results.

## Uses:

This is an excellent Mudra for enhancing one's digestive capabilities.

This Mudra causes proper and complete assimilation of the consumed food and also helps the body get rid of toxins.

# Mudras #6

## *Praanamudra / Mudra of Life*

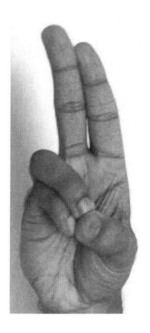

**Method:**

This Mudra is to be performed in a sitting position.

Be seated comfortably in an upright posture and concentrate on your breathing to relax.

Place your hands on your thighs with your palms facing upwards.

Touch the tip of your Thumb with the tip of your Ring finger and the tip of your Little finger.

Keep the index finger and the Middle finger straight as shown in the image.

## Duration:

This Mudra should be performed for at least 5 minutes and can be performed for 40 minutes at a stretch.

This Mudra should be performed twice a day, once in the morning and once in the evening for best results.

## Uses:

The Pranamudra is also called as the 'trigger mudra' since, when performed regularly it activates our bodies capability of self-healing

It improves the digestion and assimilation capabilities of our body, also helps our body to throw out/burn toxic fat.

An important psychological effect of this Mudra is that it imparts very good willpower to its practitioner.

# Mudras #7

## *Surabhimudra (Dhenumudra) / Mudra of Cow*

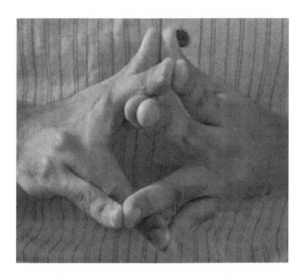

**Method:**

This Mudra is to be performed in a sitting position.

Be seated comfortably in an upright posture and concentrate on your breathing to relax.

Touch the tip of the Little finger of the left hand to the tip of the Ring finger of the right hand.

Touch the tip of the Middle finger of the left hand to the tip of the Index finger of the right hand.

Touch the tip of the ring finger of the left hand to the tip of the Little finger of the right hand.

Touch the tip of the Index finger of the left hand to the tip of the Middle finger of the right hand. (This is a bit confusing; refer to the image for clarity)

Then join the tips of both the Thumbs together and press slightly.

Hold this Mudra in front of your chest.

**Duration:**

This Mudra should be performed for at least 5 minutes and can be performed for 30 minutes at a stretch.

This Mudra should be performed twice a day, once in the morning and once in the evening for best results.

**Uses:**

This Mudra improves the digestion and assimilation capabilities of our body, along with that this Mudra has excellent positive psychological effects on our confidence.

This Mudra connects your sexual energy to your spiritual energy.

(This Mudra is extremely useful in balancing The *Vata Dosha* and also plays a pivotal role in awakening the *Manipur Chakra {Chakra of the Solar Plexus}*.)

# Mudras #8

## *Adhomukhmudra / Mudra that Faces Down*

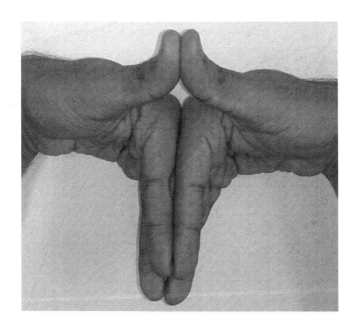

## Method:

This Mudra is to be performed in a sitting position.

Be seated comfortably in an upright posture and concentrate on your breathing to relax.

Now bring both your palms in front of you, the palms should be facing downward.

Join the tips of both your Thumbs and press slightly.

All other fingers should be pointed downwards and outstretched in such a way that all the nails are resting on each other. (refer the image)

## Duration:

It's a highly effective Mudra, also a very strong one.

Perform this Mudra for not more than 5-7 minutes at a time, and a t total of 3-4 sessions per day.

## Uses:

This Mudra is extremely effective in igniting your digestive fire and thus leading to a proper assimilation of consumed food and removal of toxins.

# Mudras #9

## *Avaahanmudra / Mudra of Calling*

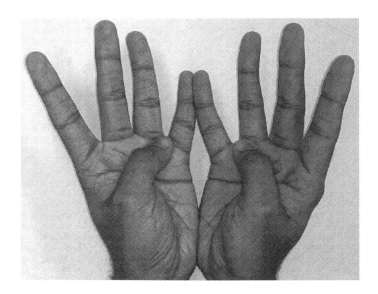

**Method:**

This Mudra is to be performed in a sitting position.

Be seated comfortably in an upright posture and concentrate on your breathing to relax.

Bring both your palms in front of your face (Palms facing you), the palms should be adjacent and the sides of the palms touching each other.

Touch the base of the Ring fingers with the tips of your Thumbs and press slightly.

The Little fingers should be touching each other at the first pad and the heel of the palms touching each other sideways.

(Refer the image)

**Duration:**

This Mudra should be performed for at least 5 minutes and can be performed for 30 minutes at a stretch.

This Mudra should be performed twice a day, once in the morning and once in the evening for best results.

**Uses:**

This Mudra Improved digestion and assimilation, and also increases your self-confidence.

# Mudras #10

## *ManipurChakramudra / Mudra of Solar Plexus Chakra*

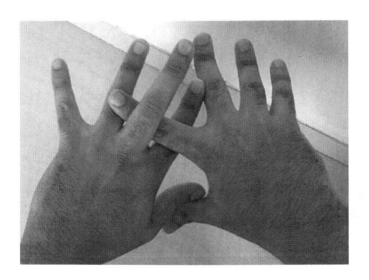

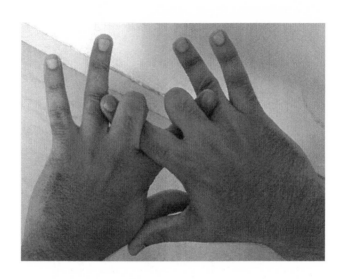

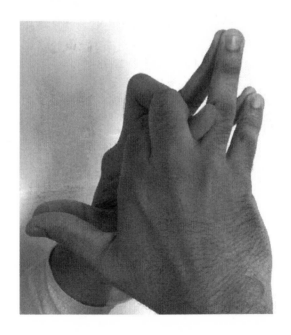

**Method:**

This Mudra is to be performed in a sitting position.

Be seated comfortably in an upright posture and concentrate on your breathing to relax.

Place your palms adjacent to each other, facing down.

Now slide your right Index finger over your left Index finger, then under the left Middle finger and then rest it over the left Ring finger. (I know it sounds very confusing, please refer the adjoining images for more clarity.)

Now curl in your left Middle finger, pressing the down the right Index finger.

The next step is to curl in the right middle finger so that it presses down the left Index finger, but see to it that the tip of the left Index finger is over the right Ring finger. (refer the image)

Now join the tips of both the Ring and Little fingers together and press slightly.

Then join the tips of both the Thumbs together and press slightly.

Hold the Mudra in front of your solar plexus.


**Duration:**

This Mudra should be performed for at least 5 minutes and can be performed for 30 minutes at a stretch.

This Mudra should be performed twice a day, once in the morning and once in the evening for best results.

**Uses:**

This Mudra Improved digestion and assimilation, and also increases your self-confidence.

This Mudra has a direct positive effect on our sexual capabilities.

# Mudras #11

## *Shankhamudra / Mudra of Conch*

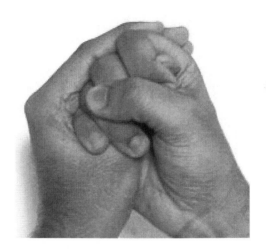

**Method:**

This Mudra is to be performed in a sitting position.

Be seated comfortably in an upright posture and concentrate on your breathing to relax.

Make a fist with your right hand.

Insert the thumb of your left hand into that fist.

Flatten the rest of the four fingers of the left hand on the fist.

Now touch the tip of the Index finger of the left hand, with the tip of the Thumb of the right hand.

This will form a *Shankha*/Conch like structure.

Refer the above image for more clarity.

Hold this Mudra in front of your chest

## Duration:

This Mudra should be performed for at least 5 minutes and can be performed for 40 minutes at a stretch.

This Mudra should be performed twice a day, once in the morning and once in the evening for best results.

## Uses:

This Mudra improves digestion and assimilation. This Mudra is extremely helpful in maintaining the health of our endocrine glands.

# Mudras #12

## *Dwitiiya Vayumudra / Mudra of Wind God II*

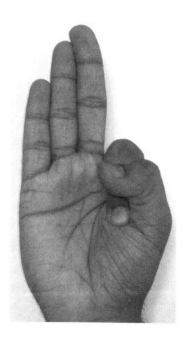

**Method:**

This Mudra can be performed while being seated, in a standing position, while walking or lying in bed.

Ideally, perform this Mudra in a seating position with your spine kept straight and upright.

Keep your palms in front of you, face up.

Touch the base of your Thumb with the tip of your Index finger and press slightly.

Now, press the bent Index finger by your Thumb. (Refer the Image)

And keep the other three fingers extended outwards.

## Duration:

This Mudra should be performed for at least 5 minutes and can be performed for 40 minutes at a stretch.

This Mudra should be performed thrice a day for best results.

## Uses:

This Mudra enhances our digestive capabilities and helps the body in throwing out the toxic fats.

# Mudras #13

## *Kangulamudra / Mudra of Hidden Potential*

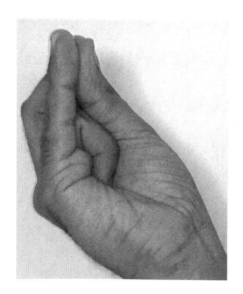

**Method:**

This Mudra is to be performed in a sitting position.

Be seated comfortably in an upright posture and concentrate on your breathing to relax.

Touch the tip of your Ring finger to the centre point of your palm and press slightly.

Join the tips of your other four fingers together and extend them as upwards as possible.

(Refer the image)

## Duration:

This Mudra should be performed for at least 5 minutes and can be performed for 45 minutes at a stretch.

This Mudra should be performed twice a day, once in the morning and once in the evening for best results.

## Uses:

This is a harmonizing Mudra which corrects any arrhythmic frequencies in your body and also improves digestion and assimilation capabilities.

# Mudras #14

## *AbhayHridaymudra / Mudra of Assured Heart*

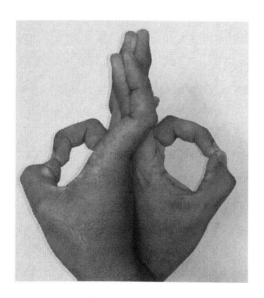

**Method:**

This Mudra is to be performed in a sitting position.

Be seated comfortably in an upright posture and concentrate on your breathing to relax.

Join your palms together as in the Indian form of salutation 'Namaste'.

Now cross the palms at your wrist, with the back of the palms facing each other and the wrist of the right hand closer to the body.

Interlock the Index, Middle and Little fingers at the tips. (Refer the image)

Join the tips of the Ring fingers and the Thumbs as shown in the image.

## Duration:

This Mudra should be performed for at least 5 minutes and can be performed for 45 minutes at a stretch.

This Mudra should be performed twice a day, once in the morning and once in the evening for best results.

## Uses:

This Mudra nourishes our Heart and is extremely helpful in enhancing our digestive capabilities.

# Mudras #15

## *Ashvaratnamudra / Mudra of Jewel among Horses*

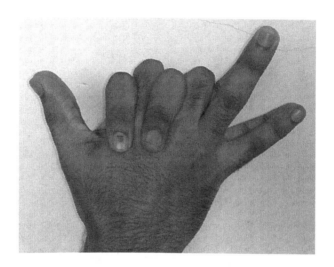

### Method:

This Mudra is to be performed in a sitting position.

Be seated comfortably in an upright posture and concentrate on your breathing to relax.

Join your hands together in front of your chest with your fingers interlaced as shown in the image.

Now extend your Thumb, Ring and Little fingers outwards.

Join the tips of the Thumbs and the Ring and Little fingers to each other as shown in the image.

**Duration:**

This Mudra should be performed for at least 5 minutes and can be performed for 45 minutes at a stretch.

This Mudra should be performed twice a day, once in the morning and once in the evening for best results.

**Uses:**

This Mudra balances the Earth, Water and Fire elements in our body at the same time increasing our digestive capabilities many folds.

# Mudras #16

## *TritiiyaVayumudra / Mudra of Wind God III*

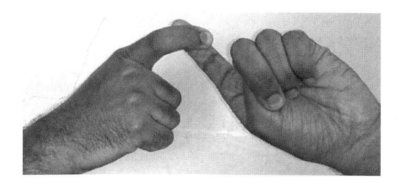

**Method:**

This Mudra is to be performed in a sitting position.

Be seated comfortably in an upright posture and concentrate on your breathing to relax.

Keep your palms in front of you, face up.

Touch the base of your Ring fingers with the tip of your Thumbs and press slightly.

Fold the Index, Middle and Ring finger over the Thumb to form a partial fist.

Now, interlock both your Index fingers at the first padding of your Index fingers as shown in the image.

## Duration:

This Mudra should be performed for at least 5 minutes and can be performed for 45 minutes at a stretch.

This Mudra should be performed twice a day, once in the morning and once in the evening for best results.

## Uses:

This is going to be the most helpful Mudra for losing weight.

This Mudra curbs and suppresses excessive craving, thus giving you a complete control over the food that tempts you into consuming more.

# Mudras #17

## *Pruthvimudra / Mudra of Earth*

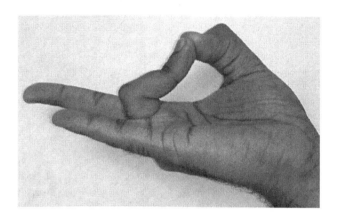

**Method:**

This Mudra is to be performed in a sitting position.

Be seated comfortably in an upright posture and concentrate on your breathing to relax.

Place your palms in your lap, facing upwards.

Join the tips of your Ring finger and Thumb together and press slightly.

Keep all the other fingers extended outwards.

## Duration:

This Mudra should be performed for at least 5 minutes and can be performed for 45 minutes at a stretch.

This Mudra should be performed twice a day, once in the morning and once in the evening for best results.


## Uses:

This Mudra enhances the Digestive and assimilation capabilities of our body.

On a psychological front, this Mudra helps us in quickly acclimatizing ourselves to a new routine. This Mudra helps us adjust with new schedule and habits.

# Mudras #18

## *Ushakaalmudra / Mudra of Morning*

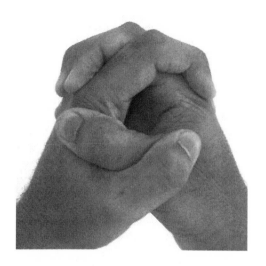

**Method:**

This Mudra can be performed while being seated, in a standing position or lying in bed.

Concentrate on your breathing to relax and feel comfortable.

Clasp both your hands together as shown in the image.

Please note that the left index figure is on top of the right index finger.

Now, bring the tips of the Index finger and Thumb of the respective hands closer, but do not let them touch, simply form an open circle.

## Duration:

This mudra should be performed for 5-10 minutes.

## Uses:

This is an extremely useful Mudra if you want to make a habit for waking up early for exercise and workout.

This mudra awakens the body and mind in morning hours.

### **NOTE

Its name literally means 'The Mudra of the Morning'; it's a Mudra which induces alertness and vitality. It is advised that this Mudra should be practiced daily when you wake up. Make a habit of performing this as a ritual when you awaken from your sleep.

### ***Important

Best results are achieved when this Mudra is performed facing the rising sun.

When you will perform this Mudra in the morning for the first time, you will feel an instant alertness induced as if you have just had a cup of espresso, this Mudra is that effective.

# Mudras #19

## *Vajramudra / Mudra of Lightning*

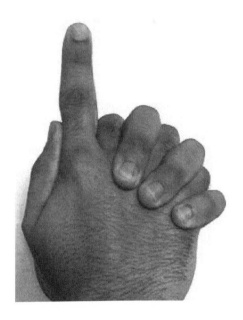

**Method:**

This Mudra can be performed while being seated, in a standing position or lying in bed.

Concentrate on your breathing to relax and feel comfortable.

First clasp your hands together.

Then, extend the Index fingers and Thumbs in an upward direction.

The outstretched index fingers should be pressing each other slightly.

Also exert slight pressure by the Thumbs on the Index fingers.

This Mudra is to be held in front of your chest, if you are lying down on your bed.

If you are sitting or standing then hold this Mudra in front of your forehead or above your head.

## Duration:

This Mudra should be performed for at least 5 minutes and can be performed for 40 minutes at a stretch.

This Mudra should be performed twice a day, once in the morning and once in the evening for best results.

## Uses:

This Mudra is known as the 'confidence booster'.

This Mudra works wonders for your willpower.

This Mudra regulates a proper flow of energy around the body.

# Mudras #20

## *Pratham Uttarbodhimudra / Mudra of Supreme Awakening I*

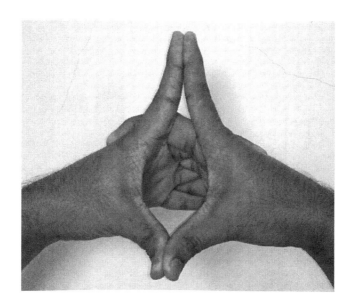

### Method:

This Mudra can be performed while being seated, in a standing position or lying in bed.

Concentrate on your breathing to relax and feel comfortable.

Interlace the fingers of both the hands together.

Now join the tips of the Index finger and the Thumbs together as shown in the image and extend the Index fingers as upwards as possible, simultaneously extending the Thumbs downwards.

(Refer the image for clarity.)

## Duration:

This Mudra should be performed for at least 5 minutes and can be performed for 40 minutes at a stretch.

This Mudra should be performed twice a day, once in the morning and once in the evening for best results.

## Uses:

This Mudra directly affects the health of the large intestine thus improving the assimilation capabilities, and on a psychological front, this Mudra enhances the willpower of the practitioner.

# Mudras #21

## *Dwitiiya Uttarbodhimudra / Mudra of Supreme Awakening II*

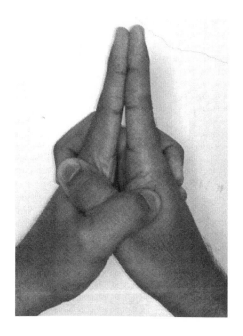

## Method:

This Mudra is to be performed in a sitting position.

Be seated comfortably in an upright posture and concentrate on your breathing to relax.

Clasp your hands together, and interlace the fingers of both the hands together.

Now join the tips of the Index finger as shown in the image and extend the Index fingers as upwards as possible,

Then cross-over the left Thumb on the right Thumb.

(Refer the image)

## Duration:

This Mudra should be performed for at least 5 minutes and can be performed for 40 minutes at a stretch.

This Mudra should be performed twice a day, once in the morning and once in the evening for best results.

## Uses:

This Mudra was used by ancient Indian Maharshi's / Yogi's for attracting inspiration and insight.

This Mudra strengthens the willpower and increases your focus towards achieving your aim.

# Forming a Routine

Every Mudra that I have mentioned in this book has to be performed for at least five minutes for best results.

But, to perform all the 21 Mudras for at least 5 minutes will eat up a little over 1 and a 1/2 hrs of your time every day and many of you might not be able to take off that much time every day from your busy schedules and chores.

Understand that <u>it is NOT a hard and fast rule that you should perform all these 21 Mudras back to back in one session</u>.

What I would suggest is, perform the first 3 Mudras every day for at least 5 times for effective weight loss, and make a habit of performing any 3 of the remaining 17 Mudras, at least twice a day.

If you follow this routine, you would successfully practice the primary Mudras regularly, and you would also, practice all the secondary Mudras throughout a week.

The beauty of Mudra Health and Healing Techniques is that Mudras can be performed at any time and place: while stuck in traffic, at the office, watching TV, or whenever you have to twiddle your thumbs waiting for something or someone.

So, please don't come up with any excuses to avoid them, Mudras are as Easy and Effortless as Weight Loss could get.

# Thank You

Thank you so much for reading my book. I hope you really liked it.

As you probably know, many people look at the reviews on Amazon before they decide to purchase a book.

If you liked the book, please take a minute to leave a review with your feedback.

60 seconds is all I'm asking for, and it would mean a lot to me.

Thank You so much.

All the best,

**Advait**

# Other Books by Advait

Mudras for Awakening Chakras: 19 Simple Hand Gestures for Awakening & Balancing Your Chakras

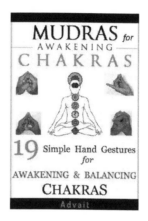

http://www.amazon.com/dp/B00P82COAY

[#1 Bestseller in 'Yoga']

[#1 Bestseller in 'Chakras']

# Mudras for Spiritual Healing: 21 Simple Hand Gestures for Ultimate Spiritual Healing & Awakening

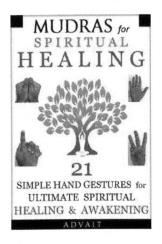

http://www.amazon.com/dp/B00PFYZLQO

Mudras for Sex: 25 Simple Hand Gestures for
Extreme Erotic Pleasure & Sexual Vitality

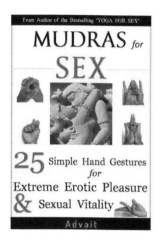

http://www.amazon.com/dp/B00OJR1DRY

Mudras: 25 Ultimate Techniques for Self Healing

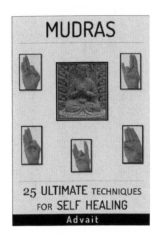

http://www.amazon.com/dp/B00MMPB5CI

Mudras of Anxiety: 25 Simple Hand Gestures for Curing Anxiety

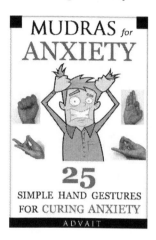

http://www.amazon.com/dp/B00PF011IU

# Mudras for a Strong Heart: 21 Simple Hand Gestures for Preventing, Curing & Reversing Heart Disease

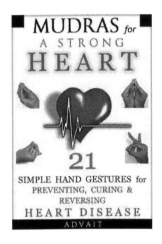

http://www.amazon.com/dp/B00PFRLGTM

Mudras for Curing Cancer: 21 Simple Hand
Gestures for Preventing & Curing Cancer

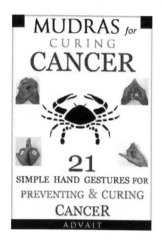

http://www.amazon.com/dp/B00PFO199M

Mudras for Stress Management: 21 Simple Hand Gestures for a Stress Free Life

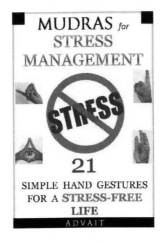

http://amazon.com/dp/B00PFTJ6OC

Mudras for Memory Improvement: 25 Simple Hand Gestures for Ultimate Memory Improvement

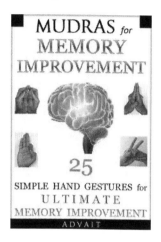

http://www.amazon.com/dp/B00PFSP8TK